Introduction

Hello Readers,

Obesity has become an enormous problem in most of the developed and developing countries today. Total number of overweight people has been increasing at an alarming rate. The simple reason of obesity is high intake of energy and its less utilization.

One simple method to reduce weight, stay fit is regular exercise but in current busy life style it is very difficult for many people to do regular exercise.

For the same reason I have written this book in which all focus has been given towards restricting intake of unwanted calorie, fat which make us overweight.

Please go through the book, follow it step by step as much as you can to get best result.

In India, there are many ashrams where this schedule is strictly followed and people across the world who have been coming to these ashrams are benefiting from this since many decades.

All the best.

Best Regards,

Narendra

For any feedback /suggestion, please email me at narendrj@gmail.com

Fastest Vegetarian/ Vegan Diet to Lose Weight– 7 Days Diet Plan To Lose 5-10 Pounds Weight

Who doesn't want to lose weight? Today almost everyone suffers from these two problems, viz. obesity and weak eye sight. We all know what obesity is but what we don't know is that it is the beginning of sickness. An obese person tends to get sick more quickly and frequently as compared to the one who is slim and healthy. The problem with obesity is that it does not come alone, instead brings in a variety of illnesses with itself. It makes your body a perfect host for diseases. Everyone wants to control their weight but does not want to do the hard work that is needed. Losing weight requires a strict and disciplined routine which needs to be followed without any IFs and BUTs.

Weight increase must be controlled from a young age itself. During the childhood stage, parents do not control their child's eating habits thinking that eating will only help in growth but thats not completely true. Diet helps in growth as it is the primary source of nourishment but it should be according to ones physical activities in day to day life. For instance, if your child plays outdoor sports regularly then his or her diet should be heavier as compared to the one that stays at home and is more into indoor activities and studies. There is a thin line between eating and over-eating. This plays an important role because parents think that only eating will help in growth whereas that is not the case.

Secondly, parents should also control the eating habits of children by controlling their craving for junk food items like noodles, pizza, chocolates, etc. Over eating occurs with the food items your child likes. Control that because such food items stick to the inner lining of stomach and intestines causing obesity and other digestive problems. Junk food items also affect ones metabolism and slows down the process of digestion which results in increase in weight.

Parents should encourage their children to do more physical activities. We already know that health is wealth and if the healthy habits are inculcated at such a young age it will stay with them forever. Parents should tell their children to drink lots of water instead of carbonated and aerated drinks. They should also inculcate the habit of personal hygiene like eating only with clean hands, keeping personal space clean etc. Such positive habits will not only make people healthy but will also keep diseases and illnesses away. To keep yourself healthy nothing is enough. Frankly speaking how much ever you do is less.

Diet Plan

The main cause of obesity is bad eating. The best way to control weight is to follow a strict diet plan. Weight loss is tough; it requires a lot of discipline along with a strict regime. You have to keep a strong will and no matter how much one tempts, have to adhere to the diet plan on a regular basis. Ensure that not even once the regime is broken. Consult any doctor or nutritionist, they too will enforce upon only one thing and that is strict following of routine. A diet plan must be accompanied with regular exercising as well. Weight loss is actually inch loss. When you exercise your mass of fat which is hollow is converted into solid muscle mass which is beneficial for the body. This results in loss of weight along with reduction in inches.

Why prefer diet plan over dieting?

Many people think that dieting is the best way of losing weight whereas this is just a misconception and that too a very common one. Dieting does not help in weight loss, on the contrary it increases weight. When a person suddenly changes his or her eating regime and starts dieting, the body thinks that it is undergoing a famine. It tries to get accustomed but before that people start eating heavily all over again. As a result of this the body thinks that the famine might come again and starts storing food. This results in the contrary effect and body gains weight instead of losing it. Our body is all about getting used to. If you'll change your eating habits out of the blue, it will only result in negative effects.

On the other hand, as discussed above, a diet plan would not only provide favorable results but also improve your health.

Indian Vegetarian Diet Plan

General Motors Inc. designed and developed a diet plan for its employees which would help them lose 5-10 Pounds of weight in a matter of 7-10 days. The Indian version of this plan is purely based on vegetarian food. You can eat non-vegetarian food too, Indian Vegetarian Diet Plan has provision for that but the most favorable results would be derived from eating vegetarian food only. It is not harmful and has better qualities than non-vegetarian food. The Indian Vegetarian Diet Plan is not only about losing weight but also about maintaining a slim and healthy body. According to this diet plan, vegetarian food is the best way of losing weight. It requires strict follow up on diet. This diet plan has various benefits, viz.

- It increases metabolism rate and improves digestion.

- It builds the habit of eating fruits and vegetables which provides all the necessary nutrients.

- One can lose as much as 10 Pounds in 7-10 days.

- Following the diet plan regularly reduces blood toxicity and provides a natural glow to skin.

- It also makes you feel energetic and light.

- It solves problems like high cholesterol, flab around stomach, thighs, sides etc.

It is an effective diet plan which will give you miraculous results in a short span of time.

Compulsory DOs and DON'Ts

The Indian version of Indian Vegetarian Diet Plan requires you to follow some instructions. These are mandatory and must be followed to the letter. **The DOs are as follows:**

- **Drink lots of water,** that is, at least 10 glasses a day. The amount should be increased to 15-20 glasses by the fifth day onwards. You'll need to drink water almost every half an hour. Water is supposed to carry minerals that keeps antibodies away. It also keeps kidneys healthy and improves the urinary system. Water provides energy and keeps body temperature normal. It boosts metabolism and reduces extra flab around your stomach. If you can drink hot water, it would be better.

- The diet plan shouldn't be begun all of a sudden. Prepare yourself from a few days before starting the diet.

- The plan is all about intake of fruits, starch, vegetables, spices and other light food items that are healthy.

- You'll also need to do an hour's exercise every alternate day to keep the system working efficiently. Although, don't do heavy exercising because it will only result in atrophy, that is, loss of muscle which is ultimately harmful for the body. So exercise less but do it on alternate days. Some Yoga will definitely bear better results.

- For quicker and better results take on the diet plan for 2 months but with a 3-4 days gap between two consecutive occasions. You need the gap for the body to cope up. But that doesn't mean you eat wholeheartedly during those gap days.

The DON'Ts include:

- No alcohol intake. You are strictly forbidden to drink alcohol for at least 10-15 days. Alcohol increases the content of uric acid which is harmful for the body. It also increases the level of toxins thereby increasing blood toxicity.

- No smoking too. We'll be removing toxins from our body and wouldn't want to add a fresh supply back to our body.

- Among beverages you are also forbidden to drink tea and coffee, since no milk and sugar is allowed. Although, you can drink black coffee and green tea.

- You are allowed to eat fruits but not allowed to drink shakes and juices. They are a strict NO for the seven days of diet plan.

- No non-veg. The Indian Vegetarian Diet Plan is strictly vegetarian. This is because non-veg food too contains toxins, fats and carbohydrates.

- No carbohydrate or fat rich food. You are not supposed to eat any junk food or items thats rich in carbohydrates and fats.

Day 1

Generally, the first day of any diet plan is the toughest because the body isn't used to eat less. This can be called as the Fruits Day as only fruits are eaten today. If you are well prepared to lose inches and maintain a fit body, this shouldn't be tough. If you are sure about taking up the challenge of losing weight, then even on the first day eating fruits must not be an issue for you. To control your craving for your favorite items try and reduce your diet from a week prior to commencement of diet plan. You can eat as many fruits you want and as many times you like. The fruits you have got to avoid are mangoes, grapes, litchis and bananas. Other than these you can eat any other fruit you want. This can be a little annoying as well as ridiculous but it has to be followed. Eat fresh fruits only and ensure they are not stale or contain pesticides.

These are specifically avoided because they contain carbohydrates which is to be avoided at all costs. You can eat fruits that have high water content and Vitamin C like oranges, lime, muskmelon, watermelon, apples etc. These fruits too have sugar but in a limited quantity as compared to the four mentioned above. The best way to eat on this day is to eat at every half an hour or so because your hunger won't be curbed only from fruits. If you'll eat in small chunks at every half an hour the craving and hunger will be minimized substantially and you'll find your tummy full throughout the day. But this is not possible with people who are working. For them control on their hunger is the only solution.

At Day 1 only fruits are eaten because it helps prepare body for the upcoming days of hardship. Try and eat juicy and pulpy fruits. If you do so, you can lose a couple of extra pounds. Do not add anything to fruits like curd, sugar, etc. Only chaat masala is allowed as a flavoring. Many would prefer taking juices instead, but eating is better. Hence, juices are strictly not allowed. Fruits have fibre which gets sieved when its juice is extracted. Fibre is good for digestive system and will be the only solid thing that can be eaten today. You are not supposed to drink any shakes because they contain milk. As written above, it is an **ONLY FRUIT DAY.**

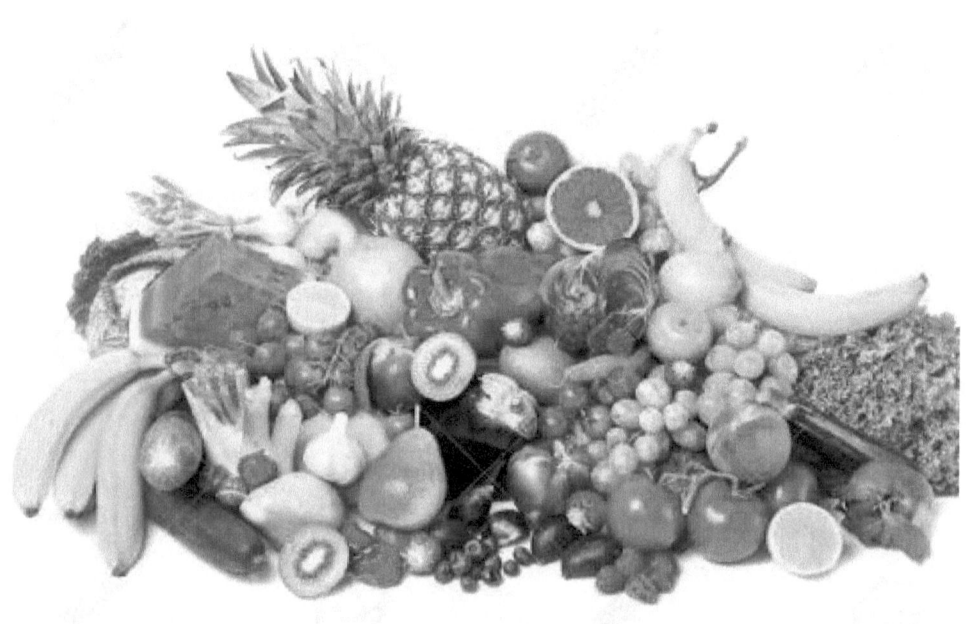

Day 2

Similar to the previous day, Day 2 is the day of veggies. On the second day you are only allowed to eat vegetables, raw or boiled, whichever you like. But no cooking, that is, use of oil, ghee, butter etc. You can eat any vegetable but try and avoid eating potatoes because they contain carbohydrates. That too the most harmful of the lot. Although, to be a little considerate, you can eat 2-3 boiled potatoes once during the day, preferably at breakfast. Other than this there is no restriction. You can add oregano seasonings, chili flakes and other spices as well. Like yesterday, Day 2 is also a calorie free day and all the necessary nutrients, viz. vitamins, minerals, fib etc. required for human body are made available through intake of vegetables. Many would want to add butter but its better to refrain from doing so because if even once the discipline is broken, it will happen repeatedly and the whole essence of the diet plan would be lost. You can also eat vegetables in the form of salad with vinegar, malt, lemon, garlic and/ or herb dressing. Although, the plain it is, the better. You can also have the GM's Wonder Soup which is made up of

- 6 large onions

- Whole tomatoes

- 2 green peppers

- 1 cabbage

- Onion soup mix

- 1 bunch of celery

- Any other vegetable as per your choice but avoid adding beans because they are high on calories

- Herbs and other flavorings as per taste

- Water

- Salt as per taste

You can have the soup as much as you want without any hesitation. The soup is full of nutrients and will boost up your metabolism.

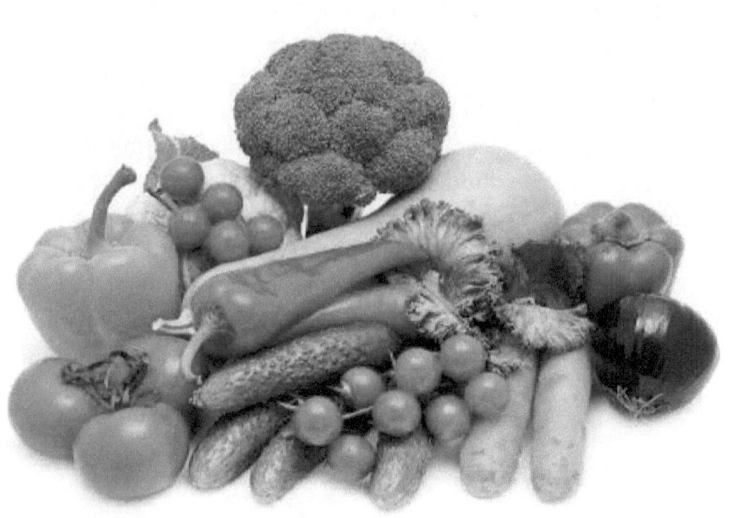

Day 3

Day 3 is dedicated to fruits and vegetables alike. There is only a slight change, that is, today you'll eat no potatoes at all. The requisite amount of carbohydrates required for energy will be provided from fruits. It can be a little boring as you haven't had anything solid since the last two days but thats the whole purpose of it. In Indian Vegetarian Diet Plan you don't stay hungry but eat only nutritious food. You can eat fruit and vegetable salad but again no oil or any other fatty substance. It will be hard but remember you'll have to lose something to gain something. Well in this case you'll lose weight which is not a loss but a definite gain. How ironical!!!

Eat unlimited fruits and veggies. Drink GM's Wonder Soup that will work as a supplement and provide energy. It will also work as a taste changer and provide you something spicier. From today onwards the excess fat will start burning. The body will start losing fat. Be happy because thats just the beginning.

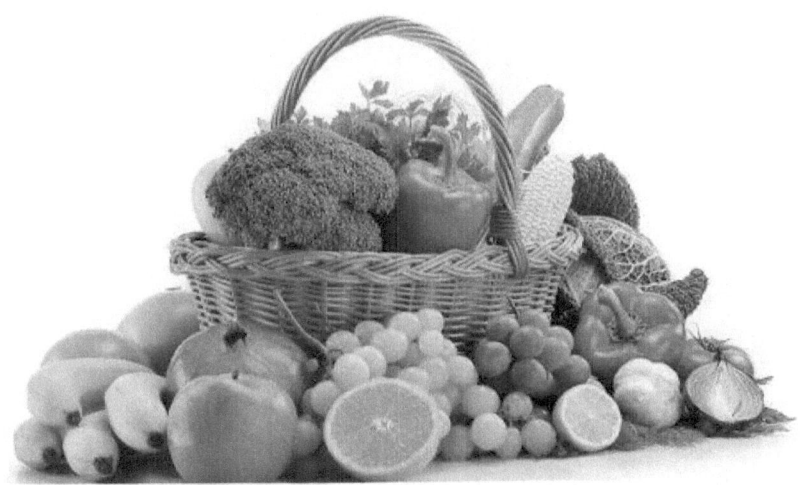

Day 4

Today you have the liberty of having some extra carbohydrates as compared to previous days. You can have 7-8 bananas which you weren't allowed to eat in the previous three days along with 3 glasses of milk. Now, the important point to remember is you need to have milk and bananas separately and not as a banana shake. You might be a little bit confused but banana and milk taken separately has a different effect on body than drinking banana shake. Banana is fatty while banana and milk eaten separately isn't. Well, this thing might be bothering you as to why are you being allowed to intake bananas when it has so many carbohydrates. The answer is that it has sodium and potassium which are important for neutralizing acidic level in your body. And the other reason is because you need adequate amount of energy to carry on with your day to day activities. Losing your weight is fine but you definitely wouldn't want to lose a week's pay.

Along with it you can also have soup but that too only once or twice. Don't have too much soup because today it is to be eaten only to pep up your taste buds.

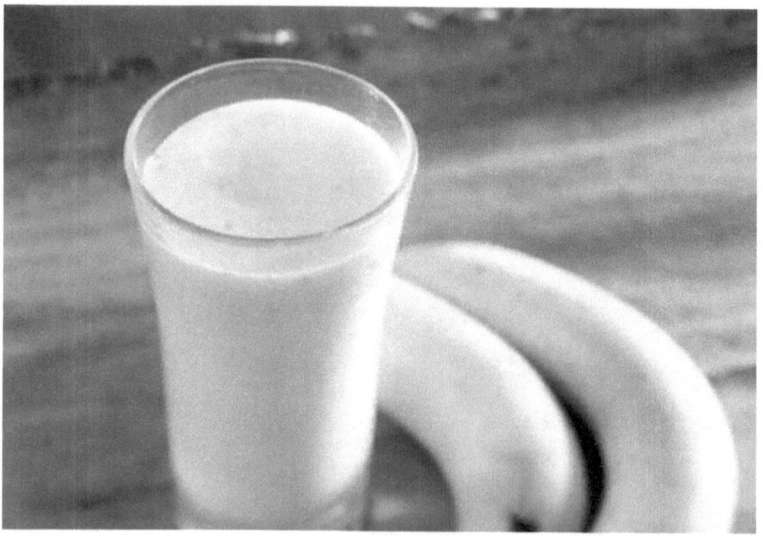

Day 5

After almost 4 days of starving yourself and living only on fruits and vegetables, today on Day 5 you'll get the chance to eat a somewhat real meal. No, don't be so happy because you ain't getting anything oily to eat. Today you'll be eating something solid, like sprouts, oatmeal, tomatoes, paneer (Cheese) , soya and similar food items that are rich in carbohydrates and proteins. This is done to prevent atrophy and maintain energy balance. You also need to improve your water intake by 25% . Unlike last four days you are not allowed to eat unlimited tomatoes or bowls of sprouts and paneer. For instance, you can only eat 6-7 tomatoes.

The tomatoes improve digestion and the water will remove the toxins thereby leveling the uric acid level in your body. Tomatoes are good for health and will help in improving metabolism. As usual you are allowed to drink soups. Drink the GM's Wonder Soup by adding your favorite veggies.

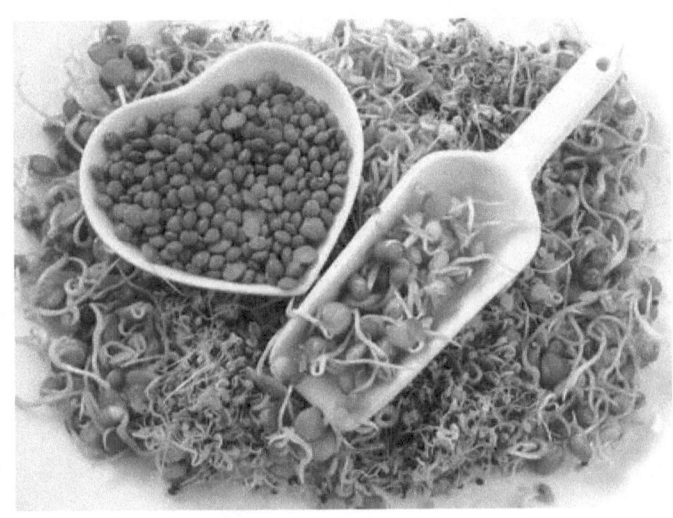

Day 6

Day 6 is not different from the previous day except that you are not allowed to eat tomatoes today. You'll have to altogether avoid them today since yesterday you ate too many of them. That was enough. Today you'll be eating baked vegetables, paneer, souls and sprouts. You also need to drink lots and lots of water as it will drain away all the toxins and other harmful substances via urinary system. Vegetables will provide necessary nutrients while paneer and sprouts will nourish the protein content. Today's diet coupled with yesterday's, will help you maintain energy levels.

You'll begin noticing the change your body has undergone in the last 5-6 days. Necessary nutrients minus fats and extra carbohydrates will ensure inch loss and depletion of flab around waist.

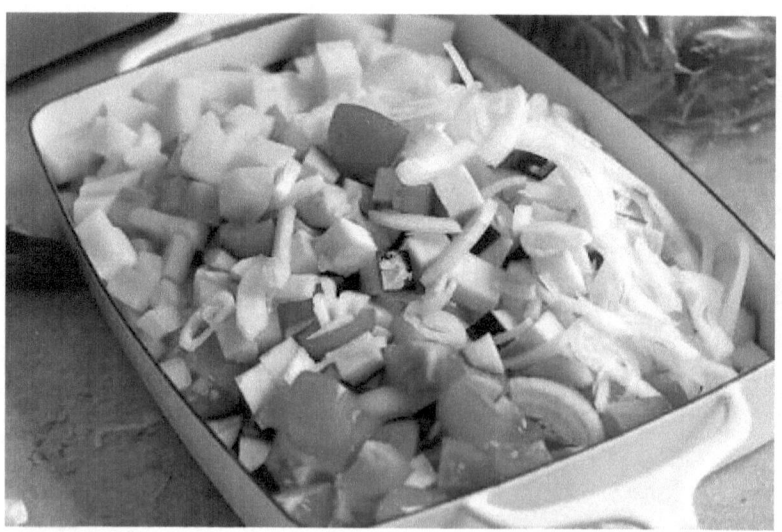

Day 7

Today is the final day of the diet plan. You'll be allowed to eat a little more than the rest of the days. This can be considered as a reward for successful completion of the Indian Vegetarian Diet Plan. Today you can eat brown rice, 1 chapati and any vegetable you want to eat. Brown rice is healthier than normal rice and contains less starch. You can also drink fresh juice. You can also cook baked vegetables and pulao out of brown rice. Try and cook food items in as less oil or ghee or butter as possible. Not to mention, but your water intake needs to at least 15-20 glasses a day.

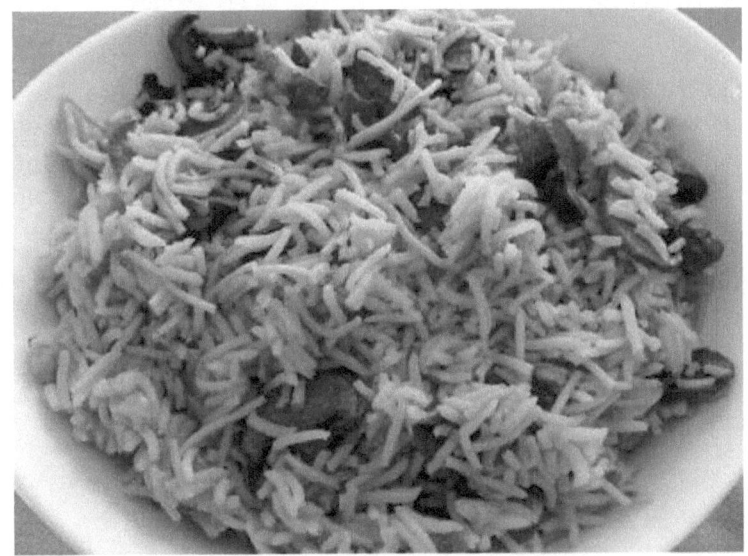

Post completion

The purpose of Indian Vegetarian Diet Plan is to regulate your eating habits and remove toxins present in your body. You have to believe in the diet plan and feel the change taking place in your body. The idea behind the diet plan is to maintain a toxic free healthy body. You can follow the diet even after completing the official seven days. Keep your eating habits post completion of Indian Vegetarian Diet Plan healthy. Intake less of fat items. Keep away from junk food. Prefer olive oil to other edible oils for cooking food as it contains less trans-fat and is healthier.

Do not change your habits back to eating unhealthy food just because you lost 5-10 Poundss of weight. Think of it as a start and maintain the diet. Eat fresh fruits vegetables and other nourishing products instead of pizza, burger, etc. Drink buttermilk, fresh fruit juices and green tea instead of carbonated drinks. Exercise regularly because only diet plans won't help you in losing weight. You'll need to exercise as well. Join a gym, play a sport, jog around, do yoga but do something as it will keep you healthy.

Eat a balanced diet like a square meal that consists of all the necessary nutrients. Eating fat and carbohydrates is not harmful unless they are completely digested. Your diet should be proportionate to your physical workout. Drink as much water as you can as it has far more benefits than healthiest of foods combined. It is important to keep the toxins out of the body because they are one of the primary reasons for making you fat.

Some recipes for the diet plan

Lets see this can be a little ironical because you'll be thinking that the plan doesn't let you eat much but still is giving you recipes. Be assured these are some of the recipes that you will require for preparation from Day 5 onwards because the previous four days were for pure raw food. Some of the recipes we'll talk about are palak paneer, sprouts, wonder soup and mushroom brown rice.

Wonder Soup

The recipe has already been given above in the Day 2 paragraph. It won't change so quickly and frequently!!! And worry not with only fruits and vegetables to eat, you'll find even wonder soup too is nothing less than elixir.

Sprouts

The best form of eating sprouts is raw without addition of any supplementary flavors. Sprouts are protein rich. It contains 4-5 forms of beans that as a whole provide a good variety of nutrients to ones body. Although, if you don't like it raw and think its tasteless, you are free to add a little olive oil, but mind you, only a little. You can also add some seasonings like oregano, chili flakes, spices and a pinch of salt, no more. To sprout lentils and beans wash them in a bowl and soak them overnight in clean water. By morning they'll be swelled. Collect the beans and wrap them inside a wet cloth. Keep them wrapped for 10-12 hours. You'll see that they have begun sprouting. The best way to eat them is raw in the form of salad by adding onions, tomatoes, lemon and salt.

Palak Paneer

You can make numerous paneer recipes like butter paneer masala, shahi paneer, paneer bhurji, paneer pasanda etc. but the most nourishing of all is palak paneer. It is not loved by many but thats the healthiest of the lot. Paneer is a source of protein and carbohydrates. It is one of those vegetarian dishes that every body builder intakes. Palak paneer has the positive qualities of palak that neutralize the oil and fat effect. It is a low calorie diet that is permitted in the Indian Vegetarian Diet Plan. It is healthy and tasty too. To make palak paneer you'll need around 2 cups of spinach, 200 grams of cubed paneer, a medium onion, 2 cloves of crushed garlic, 1/2 inch ginger, spices like garam masala, red chili powder, cumin seeds, turmeric, coriander powder and salt.

Now getting to the preparation part. Mouth already watering, eh? Clean the spinach and boil it for 3 minutes in fresh water. After that put it in ice cold water for around 5-6 minutes. In the meantime take a dry pan, heat it a little and pour one teaspoon of olive oil. Now make a paste of onion, spinach and crushed garlic. Pour it in the pan along with some cumin seeds. Fry it till it gets dark green. Now add paneer cubes to it and add one teaspoon of above mentioned spices. Add salt as per taste. Now cook it for another 5 to 10 minutes. Your palak paneer is ready to be served.

Mushroom Brown rice

Brown rice is gluten free and is healthy as compared to white rice. It is rich in fibre and is a low-calorie item. Mushroom on the other hand is rich in protein. The ingredients required to make this recipe are 1 cup of brown rice, a cup of sliced mushrooms, chopped garlic, onion, chilies, tomatoes, lettuce, turmeric powder, salt, chili powder, cumin seeds and olive oil. To prepare the recipe, boil the rice till the grains become soft. Take a fry pan and add a teaspoon of olive oil. Add cumin seeds and fry it till its dark brown. Add onion, garlic and chillies. Fry them for a minute or two. Add brown rice, mushrooms and lettuce. Fry it for sometime. Mix well and cook it for 2-3 minutes. Your savory hot dish is ready to be eaten.

Sample diet plan

Here is a sample diet chart for all of you. This will help you maintain a proper diet plan for the rest of the week. This is just a sample and can be modified as per your comfort.

Day 1

- Drink hot water in the morning. Take a heavy breakfast that consists of fruits and only fruits. Eat an apple or few slices of watermelon. You can eat any other fruit as well.

- At around 10- 10.30 you can have snacks like fruit salad. You can skip this meal if you want.

- At 12 noon again have some fruits like melon, kiwi, papaya etc. This frequent eating will keep your stomach filled and prevent craving.

- Take a late afternoon snack at around 3.30 PM. Again have a fruit or fruit salad. At this time oranges would be good.

- At 5 PM have green tea or black coffee but nothing that contains milk or carbonated water.

- Take an early dinner at 8 PM. Have a heavy dinner because it will all get digested quite soon and empty stomach would cause disruption of sleep.

- Drink lots of water throughout the day. The quantity should be at least 10 glasses a day.

Day 2

- Today is the day of veggies. Like yesterday start your morning with a glass of lukewarm water. It will improve your digestion.

- For breakfast have 2 boiled potatoes but no more. You can add chaat masala or chili powder. Mash the potato add chili powder, a pinch of salt and chaat masala.

- At 11 AM have cabbage or tomatoes or some other vegetable you are fond of.

- Drink lots of water in between and throughout the day.

- For lunch have vegetable salad and GM Wonder Soup. It will change the flavor of your mouth and sill also provide energy.

- For your evening snack, at around 4 PM have green tea or black coffee. Remember no milk products and aerated drinks.

- For dinner have salad and soup. The combination will fill your tummy and you won't have to sleep empty stomach. You may take a heavy dinner if you like.

Day 3

- As usual begin your day with a glass of hot water. Try and gradually increase the intake of water. It is important to remove toxins from your body and water is the best medium.

- For breakfast have a combination of fruits and vegetables. No potatoes today. Have tomatoes if you like.

- For the 11 AM brunch have GM's Wonder soup and add your favorite vegetables to it. Have a fruit salad if you like. An orange or a few slices of watermelon would be better choice.

- At lunch have salads and drink soup.

- Repeat the same meal for the evening snack at 4 pm. Eat pear or pineapple or a few slices of melon. Alternate veggies to ensure you don't get bored.

- For dinner have a fruit and vegetable salads. Take a cup of black coffee or green tea if you have had enough of GM's Wonder soup.

Day 4

- Drink hot water, first thing in the morning.

- At breakfast have 2-3 bananas and a glass of milk.

- At 11 AM have have vegetable soup and some fruits. 1 banana too would do along with pear, apple or pineapple.

- For lunch have another 2 bananas and a glass of milk. If you want you can have vegetable salad as well.

- For evening snack have green tea of black coffee. Even though you are allowed to drink milk today but don't use it to make tea or coffee.

- Have a heavy dinner. Eat 2-3 bananas and a glass of milk. Along with this you can have fruit or vegetable salad or a combination of both.

- You need to gradually increase you water intake to 12 glasses a day.

Day 5

- Begin your day with a glass of hot water. Today you'll need to have at least 15 glasses of water. Don't have it before half an hour of eating a meal.

- Have a couple of tomatoes, kidney beans or sprouts. Garnish it with lettuce, lemon, salt and pepper. You can also have oatmeal if you want. Its healthy and nutritious.

- For afternoon brunch have a cup of curd or tofu.

- At lunch have brown rice, palak paneer and sprouts.

- In the evening have some more sprouts and a cup of green tea or black coffee, whichever you like.

- At dinner have a couple of bowls of vegetable soup, some more sprouts and fruits if you like. Have some palak paneer if you want.

Day 6

- The food schedule will be similar to yesterday except for some minor changes. As usual begin your day with hot water. You'll need to drink lots and lots of water.

- At breakfast have sprouts and a bowl of boiled veggies. Add some salt and pepper to make it tasty.

- Since no tomatoes today, have soup and a bowl of fresh fruits for brunch. Have as much soup as you like.

- At lunch have a cup of mushroom brown rice. Also, eat a medium bowl of vegetable salad with it.

- In the evening have green tea or black coffee along with a bowl of sprouts.

- At night have a bowl of baked or boiled veggies. Have some fruits and a bowl of sprouts.

Day 7

- Today is the last day but you don't have to be too happy about it because you'll control your diet even after the plan officially ends. Drink a glass of water after waking up. The water intake today must be between 15-20 glasses.

- At breakfast have fresh fruits like watermelon, orange and pineapple. Some juicy fruits in the morning will be good for your health.

- At noon have a glass of fresh fruit juice along with a bowl of sprouts. You can complement it with some strawberries, if you like.

- At lunch have boiled veggies and a bowl of brown rice cooked with mushrooms.

- In the evening you can have fruits along with green tea or black coffee.

- At dinner, have GM's Wonder soup and vegetable salad. Have some sprouts too.

If you'll follow this diet plan or something similar to it you can easily go through the seven days. The success of the diet plan depends upon you. You'll need to keep yourself motivated throughout the diet plan. Its the perception that matters. Everything related to our body is about believing. A theory says that it is not the medicine that cures a person but his or her belief that he or she will be cured through the intake of that medicine. Keep a strong head and believe in the while thing. Your belief will seek better results. You can have the diet with non-vegetarian food items too but vegetarian food and weight loss goes hand in hand. It will give you the best weight loss solutions.

Try and keep up the good eating habits even after the diet plan is completed. Nourish your body with healthy and nutritious food instead of toxins like alcohol, junk food etc. Keep the blood toxicity neutral and drink lots and lots of water. It will drain every ounce of toxic elements from your body. It will rejuvenate your organs and make them healthy. So eat healthy and stay healthy.

I hope I was able to provide step by step easy to follow guide in achieve you dream goal of achieving and maintaining your ideal body weight.

If you have any feedback/suggestion, please feel free to mail at narendrj@gmail.com.

If you like this, I request you to please checkout my other book which will help you to live a healthy life naturally

https://www.amazon.in/dp/B01KDWYVOK

Warm Regards,

Narendra

New Delhi

www.ingramcontent.com/pod-product-compliance
Lightning Source LLC
Chambersburg PA
CBHW050530290526
45786CB00007B/2762